MW00618874

FOR OPTIMAL HEALTH

You may require more of one single nutrient than your body can manufacture. Mountain climbers, marathon runners and even commuters can gain endurance and muscle with octacosanol. Carnitine has been found to improve neuro-muscular diseases; taurine helps prevent gallstones and the loss of potassium and calcium from the heart. Glucomannan suppresses appetite. It also helps blood fat problems and normalizes blood sugar. These "accessory" concentrated foods represent the new explosion of information, the important happening now going on in *individual* nutritional therapy and research.

ABOUT THE AUTHOR AND EDITORS

Jeffrey Bland, Ph.D., is a promoter of good health — whether he is teaching, practicing, lecturing or writing, he is actively committed to the idea that the relationship between health and lifestyle when properly revised leads to longer, healthier lives and more productive contributions to the survival of our species. A Ph.D. in biochemistry, he is Professor of Nutritional Biochemistry at the University of Puget Sound, Director of the Bellevue Redmond Medical Laboratory and the dedicated advocate of healthful common sense from the lecture platform primarily to physicians, dentists and other scientists. His latest book is *Your Health Under Siege* and he has also authored many magazine articles.

Richard A. Passwater, Ph.D., is one of the most called-upon authorities for information relating to preventive health care. A noted biochemist, he is credited with popularizing the term "supernutrition" largely as a result of having written two bestsellers on the subject — *Supernutrition: Megavitamin Revolution* and *Supernutrition for Healthy Hearts*. His other books include *Easy No-Flab Diet*, *Cancer and Its Nutritional Therapies*, and the recently published *Selenium as Food & Medicine*. He has just completed a new book on *Hair Analysis* with Elmer M. Cranton, M.D.

Earl Mindell, R.Ph., Ph.D., combines the expertise and working experience of a pharmacist with extensive knowledge in most of the nutrition areas. His book *Earl Mindell's Vitamin Bible* is now a million-copy bestseller; and his more recent *Vitamin Bible for Your Kids* may very well duplicate his first *Bible's* publishing history. Dr. Mindell's popular *Quick & Easy Guide to Better Health* was just published by Keats Publishing.

Volume 2

OCTACOSANOL, CARNITINE AND OTHER "ACCESSORY" NUTRIENTS

MAKE THE MOST OF YOUR HEALTH WITH NUTRIENTS YOUR OWN BODY NEEDS

by Jeffrey Bland, Ph.D.

Keats Publishing, Inc. New Canaan, Connecticut

Octacosanol, Carnitine and Other "Accessory" Nutrients is not intended as medical advice. Its intention is solely informational and educational. Please consult a medical or health professional should the need for one be warranted.

OCTACOSANOL, CARNITINE AND OTHER "ACCESSORY" NUTRIENTS

Copyright © 1982 by Keats Publishing, Inc.

All Rights Reserved

No part of this book may be copied or reproduced in any form without the written consent of the publisher.

ISBN: 0-87983-316-5

Printed in the United States of America

Good Health Guides are published by Keats Publishing, Inc.
27 Pine Street (Box 876)
New Canaan, Connecticut 06840

Contents

Contents

Volume 2
OCTACOSANOL, CARNITINE AND OTHER "ACCESSORY" NUTRIENTS

INTRODUCTION

As was pointed out in Volume I of this series on accessory food factors in clinical nutrition, these nutrients are substances that may be manufactured within the human body and therefore are not considered essential nutrients as such. (The term "essential" means that the substance is not manufactured within the human body, but is necessary for survival and so must be gotten from the diet.) The use of these accessory factors such as carnitine and taurine, both of which are manufactured within the body, is for specific therapeutic need in the individuals who are incapable of manufacturing the amount necessary for optimal health. Concentration of these principles from natural food sources can then lead to the formulation of specific food supplements for individuals who require more of the specific agent than they can manufacture. This can be called nutritional pharmacology, a new branch of clinical nutrition that recognizes the function of certain food concentrates in the management of specific individuals.[1]

A recent review article by Bessman[2] has pointed out that even amino acids generally considered "nonessential" for most individuals may be essential for a few people who do not have adequate ability to manufacture them within their own bodies. Bessman calls this the Justification Theory that indicates, on the basis of an individual's unique genetic nature when a nonessential nutrient may become an essential nutrient. The use of this accessory food factor in supplemental doses becomes "essential" for that individual's good health.

Four such examples of these therapeutic nutrients are octacosanol, carnitine, taurine and glucomannan. None of these substances will be found listed in the tables of essential nutrients for humans; however, each has found specific therapeutic value in certain individuals. It should be remembered that *nu-*

trition is for real individuals. The statistical human or the average man is of little value in assessing the need for therapeutic nutrition.

Historically, the nutritionists' interest has been the study of the effects of essential nutrients in food on the biochemical and physiological function of humans. In this volume, this interest has been expanded to include accessory substances within foods which may be used therapeutically to help specific individuals with a pharmacological need.[3]

OCTACOSANOL

For millennia, early humans ate diets high in unrefined grains which were rich in unsaturated oils, vegetable fats and waxes. As our diets grew more processed and refined, many of these oils in their natural state were removed. As a result of these dietary changes, animal fat began to replace the natural oils and fat principles found in whole wheat, rye, corn and millet. Wheat germ was one of the foods highest in unsaturated oil content, as well as a rich source of vitamin E and protein. In the 1930s a commercial process to extract the oils from wheat germ was developed and when these oils were administered in the diets of human volunteers, improvement in endurance and stamina was observed. Studies by William Smiley[4] and Charles White[5] in the 1950s indicated reduced oxygen stress and quickened reaction time in exercise studies done on trained and untrained individuals. Later Ershoff and Levin found a beneficial effect of an unidentified factor in wheat germ oil on the swimming performance of guinea pigs.[6] This observation set the biochemists to work to determine what the principle or principles in wheat germ oil might be that helped improve exercise tolerance. At first it was thought that it might be vitamin E, but later it was concluded that the observed beneficial effects were not due to vitamin E. Studies on animals confirmed that there was a significant difference in the therapeutic benefit of vitamin E and wheat germ oil, with the wheat germ oil principle being superior for improving endurance.[7]

The chemical principles of wheat germ oil were finally established to include essential fatty acids such as linoleic acid, vitamin E, and a high boiling residue made up of long-chain alcohols and plant sterols. The long-chain alcohols included octacosanol, triacontanol, tetracosanol and hexacosanol. A commercial process was developed and patented by Ezra Levin to extract these long-chain alcohols from wheat germ oil, and human studies were started by Dr. Thomas Cureton on the effect of these substances on improving stamina and exercise tolerance. The patent held by Levin (patented April 24, 1962, No. 3,031,376) led to the production of a wheat germ oil concentrate high in several long-chain alcohols and neutral plant sterols.

Clinical Utility: Studies by Alfin-Slater indicated that this unidentified complex mixture of substances was capable of decreasing blood cholesterol.[8] Recent work by Vahouny and Kritchevsky[9] seems to indicate that this is a result of the high plant sterol content of beta-sitosterol in wheat germ oil which blocks excessive blood cholesterol.

Cureton found that factors in this wheat germ oil concentrate which improved endurance seemed to be related to octacosanol, the 28 carbon straight chain, saturated alcohol.[10] Work by Farrell in animals confirmed that these long-chain alcohols improved oxygen utilization.[11]

The studies on humans who were administered doses of this concentrate orally, equivalent to 1000 micrograms of octacosanol and 2000 micrograms of the other naturally occurring long-chain alcohols, indicated:

    1. Improved muscle glycogen storage

2. Stability of basal metabolic rate under stress
3. Reduced high altitude stress
4. Improved reaction time
5. Reduced oxygen debt
6. Improved endurance.

Commercial Process: These clinical studies were all done with the natural concentrate from wheat germ oil, manufactured by the Levin process (Viobin Corporation). Recently, purified octacosanol has become available from nonwheat-germ sources. These products make label claim of very high octacosanol content, but it should be pointed out that these are not the products used by Cureton in his clinical studies. The usefulness of the wheat germ oil concentrate may very well be due to its complex synergistic mixture of various alcohols and plant sterols. Highly purified, petrochemically originated octacosanol cannot offer this complex mixture of natural materials. The burden of proof for clinical usefulness of these pure octacosanol products is on the shoulders of the manufacturers. Failure to achieve the desired results with octacosanol concentrates may be due to the product quality and composition. The naturally derived wheat germ oil concentrate remains the only clinically proven substance that has ergogenic activity (improvement of oxygen utilization when exercising).

It is possible to get these principles from whole grains, but it should be pointed out that ten pounds of whole wheat are concentrated to give 1000 micrograms equivalent of octacosanol under the Levin process.

In sum, the therapeutic use of wheat germ oil concentrate has support in clinical studies for improved exercise tolerance, reduced blood cholesterol, improved oxygen utilization, and as a neuromuscular factor to prohibit muscle pain after exercise.[12] Muscular dystrophies and other neuromuscular disorders have proven responsive to wheat germ oil concentrate.[13] The wheat germ oil concentrate used in Dr. Thomas Cureton's studies which indicated the positive effect of this substance on exercise and oxygen utilization can be considered the application of therapeutic nutrition. It is not a supplement required necessarily by everyone, but its effect in improving oxygen utilization and in lowering blood cholesterol may be most helpful for those individuals who experience muscle pain after exercise, poor exercise tolerance or lowered endurance.

CARNITINE

Dietary Sources and Function: Carnitine is an unusual amino acid that is biosynthesized in the liver of humans and is found highest in muscle and organ meats in the human diet. Carnitine is not found in vegetable sources. In human metabolism it is utilized as a material which transfers fatty acids across the membranes of the mitochondria (which are like the lungs of the cell) where they can be used as a source of fuel to generate energy. In the absence of proper carnitine levels within the cell, the fatty acids are poorly metabolized and can build up within the cell or the surrounding medium, thereby leading to elevated blood fat and triglyceride levels.[14]

Carnitine has been found to have an important regulatory effect upon fat metabolism in heart and skeletal muscles. The administration of carnitine in tissue culture has been shown to stimulate fat metabolism and encourage the clearance of triglycerides and fatty acids.[15]

Carnitine is not a vitamin, because it can be manufactured in the human body, but it is somewhat like the relationship of niacin to tryptophan.[16] It is well known that niacin can be partially manufactured from tryptophan, but not in adequate amounts to prevent a niacin deficiency, called pellagra. Carnitine, likewise is manufactured in the body from the amino acids lysine and methionine, but again not at levels adequate to meet the needs of all individuals, particularly if they are on a low lysine or methionine diet. It should be pointed out that lysine and methionine are both essential amino acids found in adequate levels in high quality protein, but which may be deficient in unbalanced vegetable protein. The reliance upon a single vegetable protein family such as wheat, soy or corn could lead to specific deficiencies of lysine or methionine and could contribute to an imbalance in the manufacture of carnitine. This may explain why some vegetarians who are on poorly balanced vegetarian diets have elevated blood fats, such as triglycerides, because of carnitine insufficiency.

There has also been found a considerable difference in the level of need for carnitine between men and women. Men have higher blood carnitine than women, and high levels of carnitine are found in the epididymis of the testes in men.[17] The spermatazoa from lysine-depleted animals became infertile due to potential carnitine insufficiency. This is the first tissue to show deficiencies in animals that have been deprived of carnitine or lysine. Adequate levels of carnitine are necessary for energy metabolism within the sperm for proper motility and fertility.[18]

The synthesis of carnitine from lysine and methionine necessitates vitamin C. The role of vitamin C in the manufacture of carnitine is similar to the role that vitamin C plays in the manufacture of hydroxyproline, an amino acid used in the manufacture of collagen, a connective tissue. Working with vitamin C in the manufacture of carnitine are vitamin B6, niacin, lysine and methionine. Low levels of vitamin C intake have also been indicated to produce symptoms of carnitine deficiency, and this is why scurvy may be associated with a high level of blood fat.[19]

Although carnitine has not been recognized as a vitamin, it may be required by newborns as a vitamin, because their biosynthetic machinery is late to develop and may be unavailable for proper carnitine biosynthesis. There seem to be genetic limitations on the ability of some individuals to synthesize carnitine from lysine or methionine, and therefore in these individuals carnitine may be an essential nutrient.[20]

Clinical Reports of Deficiency: Engel and Angelini reported the first carnitine deficiency in humans in 1972.[21] In this case, they report infiltration of the liver with fat and depressed muscle carnitine levels with generalized spleen and liver enlargement and muscle wasting. Human carnitine deficiencies, which have been identified since 1972, range from actual deficiencies of carnitine due to dietary and biosynthetic unavailability to transport problems of carnitine as it relates to the inability of individuals to transport carnitine in their blood to the cells of need.

Chapoy and coworkers recognized a carnitine deficiency which resembles Reyes syndrome.[22] The case history was that of a 6-month-old boy who had heart failure, an enlarged liver, gross retardation, infections of the respiratory tract, with fatty liver and low liver carnitine levels. After a number of years of not knowing what was wrong with the boy it was finally recognized that he might be suffering from a carnitine deficiency. He was then given 4000 mg per day of carnitine and showed remarkable improvement almost immediately. Over a period of two years his health changed for the better and it was determined that he was suffering from a defect in the enzyme responsible for the manufacture of carnitine from lysine and methionine. The effective treatment of this youngster led to the mobilization of fat from the heart and muscle, a diminution of the heart size, improved muscle strength and improved neurological function.

Therapeutic Use of Carnitine: The most exciting recent advances in the use of carnitine in clinical nutrition is as an agent to improve fat metabolism and to reduce blood triglycerides when 1000 to 3000 mg of dl-carnitine are administered daily.[23] Elevated triglycerides can lead to increased risk to small vessel diseases, such as poor circulation in the hands and feet, kidney problems and the inability to walk without pain, called claudication. The management of this problem by utilizing a lower fat diet with lower sugar and increased carnitine as a supplement has effectively reduced triglycerides in patients who have blood triglyceride levels of 800 to 1000 mg/100 ml (normal range less than 150 mg/100 ml).

Neuromuscular diseases such as certain myopathies or problems with the heart, muscular dystrophy, myotonic dystrophy and limb-girdle muscular dystrophy have all been suggested to be aided or improved by administration of carnitine as a supplement. There is some indication that these neuromuscular diseases lead to an increased loss of carnitine in the urine and therefore may require higher levels for adequacy.[24]

Carnitine has also been found to be helpful in those people who want to improve fatty acid metabolism due to metabolic obesity problems. Many weight-loss diets cause a problem called ketosis which is the accumulation of ketone bodies or fat waste products in the blood. These ketones can cause the blood to become acid and lead to the loss of calcium, magnesium and potassium in the urine. Ketosis when uncontrolled in poor weight-loss diets or diabetes can be life-threatening. The use of carnitine in therapeutic doses as a food supplement can encourage the proper metabolism of fats and prevent ketones from building up in people who are susceptible to ketosis.[25] Prevention of ketosis can be the difference between a poorly controlled and well-controlled weight-loss diet.

The future of this accessory food factor in clinical nutrition is very rich, and as studies are made to indicate specifically the various forms of neuromuscular and fatty acid diseases that may respond to supplements of carnitine, its application in health care will increase.

TAURINE

Dietary Sources and Function: Taurine is another amino acid which is manufactured in the human body and therefore is not considered an essential nutrient. It is known to be a neurotransmitter in the central nervous system of humans and other animals, but it has only been identified as an essential nutrient in cats. Taurine is found only in animal products and not in vegetable protein sources. It is a sulfur amino acid derivative, and this may indicate why cats on soy protein diets or heavy vegetable-based protein diets may develop certain types of neurological and behavioral changes.[26]

Taurine was first derived from ox bile, where it is found in high concentration. In the human it is biosynthesized from the amino acids cysteine and methionine, which are two sulfur amino acids found in high quality dietary protein. Vegetarians who are on imbalanced dietary proteins of lower quality may have difficulty manufacturing adequate levels of taurine.

Most taurine in humans is synthesized in the liver, and there is only a limited ability for this synthesis. Vitamin B6 has been found necessary for the manufacture of taurine in the liver from methionine and cysteine.

Women may have much more need for taurine in the diet than men since the female hormone estradiol is found to inhibit the synthesis of taurine in the liver. Certain estrogenic hormone substances when given to women may therefore increase the inhibition of taurine synthesis and require even more dietary intake.[27]

Taurine is found in the brain as a neurotransmitter working along with the other neuroinhibitory transmitters gamma aminobutyric acid (GABA) and glycine. Large oral doses of taurine have been found to increase growth hormone in animals.

Taurine also conjugates chemically with bile acids in the liver. This seems to be very important for the maintenance of proper bile composition and for keeping cholesterol soluble. The liver is the only tissue where taurine has metabolized, although there have been high levels found in the retina, brain and heart.[28]

Taurine works by itself as a single amino acid substance and it has been found to be concentrated in the pineal and pituitary glands in higher levels when the individual has been exposed to full spectrum light.[29] A deficiency of exposure to the near ultraviolet portion of the spectrum (which occurs when an individual is only exposed to fluorescent lights or incandescent bulbs) may lead to impaired concentration of the neurotransmitter taurine in the pineal and pituitary glands.

Increased urinary spill of taurine has been found when individuals have been placed under stress. Taurine works with zinc in the eyes, and deficiencies of taurine have led to functional impairment of vision well before there was an actual structural alteration of the eye.[30] In animals, depletion of taurine occurs slowly, but eventually leads to blindness. Between 25 and 90 percent of the taurine in the body is conjugated to bile salts, and this makes the bile less lithogenic or prevents cholesterol gallstones.

Taurine is the second most abundant amino acid in human milk, and infants may need taurine above what is found in cow's milk or a soy formula. Being without it may lead to growth depression, which has been shown in many primates such as monkeys and apes.[31]

Neurological Disorders and Taurine: Taurine's role in the central nervous system is that of an inhibitory neurotransmitter. Deficiencies of taurine may produce memory loss, although the results are not very reproducible in this area. The brain is in subtle balance between the messages coming from the neuroexcitatory transmitters, such as the serotonin and dopamine family, and the neuroinhibitory transmitters, such as GABA and taurine. When there is a deficiency of the neuro-inhibitory transmitters, there is an over-excitation of certain portions of the brain which may lead to convulsions. Because of this observation, Huxtable and Barbeau attempted to use oral doses of taurine in the treatment of epilepsy or as an anti-convulsant in drug toxicities.[32] They found that taurine influenced the movement of calcium ions in the brain, and that the observed anticonvulsant effects of taurine may be a result of this biochemical effect. Taurine undoubtedly serves both as a neurotransmitter and a neuromodulator substance in the management of central nervous system function.

Potassium-Sparing Effects of Taurine: An additional important role that taurine plays is to spare the loss of potassium from the heart muscle. Recent evidence indicates that taurine may be the critical substance in the osmotic regulation of both calcium and potassium concentrations within the heart muscle and in preventing potassium or calcium wasting, particularly during times of weight-loss dieting.[33] It is well known that the heart irregularities in a number of people who were on the liquid protein diets a few years back were very similar to those produced during times of potassium depletion. This seemed unusual, since many of the people on these diets were actually on potassium supplementation. Follow-up studies indicated that many of the liquid protein weight-loss products were low in the amino acids cysteine or methionine, and thereby may have led to the inability of the heart muscle to retain potassium and to the observed heart problems.[34] It can be seen then that proper amounts of taurine seem essential to prevent potassium and calcium loss from the heart during bio-chemical stress on a weight-loss diet. Those proteins which are rich in the sulfur amino acids should especially be supplied at those times to avoid taurine deficiency.

Taurine and Nutritional Individuality: Taurine has also been found to resemble the effect of insulin on blood sugar. It seems to promote the proper regulation of blood sugar in the individual who may be insulin insufficient.[35]

Vitamin A and vitamin E deficiency lead to increased taurine excretion with greater need for intake. Recently these vitamins have been found to play some role in the management of muscular dystrophy, although this work is still in the early stages of clinical investigation.[36]

The whole array of metabolic genetic problems associated with sulfur amino acid metabolism, of which many are known, may indicate a dietary increased need for taurine. Conditions such as homocystinuria or cystathioninuria, which are known to be vitamin B6 dependent, may also indicate the need for supplemental taurine.

Lastly, taurine has been intimated to be a limiting nutrient in some forms of mental retardation, such as in Down's syndrome. Studies are now under way to look at the effect on intelligence quotient in those Down's syndrome children who are supplemented with taurine. This accessory food factor may work along with the B-complex vitamins and vitamins C and E in the improvement of intelligence in mentally retarded individuals.[37]

Taurine is one of those remarkable accessory food factors whose therapeutic use is just now beginning to be understood. Its panoramic effects cover functional applications from the management of some forms of epilepsy to the prevention of potassium and calcium loss from the heart muscle to improved bile composition and the prevention of gallstones. It should be recalled that dietary taurine comes exclusively from animal products, and is related to the sulfur amino acids; therefore, metabolic defects in the metabolism of the sulfur amino acids may lead to insufficiencies of taurine and require augmented dietary intake.

GLUCOMANNAN

The symptoms of tiredness, mood swings, shakiness, dizziness, sweating, inability to concentrate or muscle weakness before or after meals have all been associated with a condition called hypoglycemia, or low blood sugar. These manifestations of low blood sugar can be amplified by individuals who consume the average American diet, which is very high in sugar, low in complex starches from whole grains and beans, and high in fat.[38]

The consumption of diets that are high in refined carbohydrates can stimulate the pancreas to secrete excessive insulin and cause a blood sugar rebound which leads to the low blood sugar condition called hypoglycemia. A more severe medical problem of a similar nature occurs when the pancreas is unable to secrete enough insulin in response to the sugar in the diet, or the carbohydrate load or the cells of the body become insensitive to insulin. This leads to elevated blood sugar, or hyperglycemia (diabetes). Both hypoglycemia and hyperglycemia are irritated and amplified when the diets are high in substances which release sugar into the blood quickly after eating. This is why diets high in sugar put a stress on the pancreas and, in fact, encourage blood sugar abnormalities.[39]

Recently, it has been found that constituents within the diet which can slow the release of sugar into the blood from the starches or sugars in the diet will diminish the stress on the pancreas, smooth the blood sugar curve, and therefore avert hypoglycemic or hyperglycemic rebound effects. Dr. James Anderson, at the University of Kentucky Medical School, has developed a diet he uses with diabetic patients to help normalize their blood sugar.[40] Using this type of diet, which Dr. Anderson calls the HCF diet, or high complex carbohydrate, high fiber diet, he has been able to reduce the daily need for insulin in diabetics by as much as twenty or more units.

The most recent finding, relating to dietary improvement in the management of blood sugar, has been the suggestion that other fibrous materials which are called dietary gums are even more important in flattening the blood sugar curve than standard wheat, oat, corn or rice bran fiber. Dr. David Jenkins has shown that gum guar is extremely important when combined with the meal in promoting proper blood sugar regulation and slowing the time of release of sugar from the diet into the bloodstream, thereby putting less demand on the pancreas.[41] This observation was confirmed in a study done by Dr. Goulder, in which he showed that patients who were insulin-requiring diabetics could produce a 20 percent decrease in elevation of blood sugar after a meal by including guar in the form of a guar-enriched bread with each meal.[42] This opened the door for explorations of other gums, which would be equally or more valuable in normalizing blood sugar, slowing down the release of sugar into the blood after a meal and encouraging proper blood fat composition.

These investigations determined that a substance derived from the tuber Amorphophallus plant, Konjac mannan, which has been called "glucomannan," had such beneficial properties. Glucomannan is an unabsorbable gum material which has been shown to have one of the most significant impacts upon normalizing blood sugar of any of the gums explored so far. Glucomannan is composed of two sugars—glucose and mannose—which are attached together in long chains in an unabsorbable form, while guar gum is composed of the sugars galactose and mannose in an unabsorbable form. Glucomannan is known to be a commonly used Japanese food-stuff, which is generally taken in jelled form and which can make a liquid into a solid at room temperature with as little as one percent by weight inclusion in the liquid. In a clinical trial of the effect that glucomannan had on normalizing blood sugar, thirteen diabetic patients were supplemented with three and a half to seven grams of glucomannan daily for three months.

Their mean serum cholesterol was reduced by 11 percent and fasting blood sugar in the diabetic men fell by 30 percent. In some patients taking glucomannan, insulin could be completely withdrawn and was no longer needed.[43]

The mechanism of the action of glucomannan is thought to relate to its ability to increase the stickiness of the food being digested and to prevent the quick release of sugar into the bloodstream, or to slow gastric emptying, acting as a barrier to the diffusion of the sugar materials into the blood.

When five healthy men underwent an oral glucose tolerance test with and without supplementation with glucomannan, significant changes in their blood sugar responses were observed. In these normal, healthy individuals glucomannan reduced blood glucose by 8 percent at 30 minutes and insulin need by 13 percent in the same period of time. It is clear that glucomannan may be a very powerful adjunct dietary agent which facilitates normalization of blood sugar after a meal and helps improve blood fats such as cholesterol and triglycerides. Being noncaloric and nondigestible, it can increase the volume of the partially digested food material, thereby producing some appetite suppression without adding calories, so it may also prove useful as an adjunct in weight-loss diets.

There seems to be no known adverse side effects from the inclusion of glucomannan in the diet. The only problem is palatability; it does considerably increase the stickiness of the diet. When put into liquids, it will cause thickening of the liquid if it is not consumed rapidly after being stirred in. Glucomannan is a virtually tasteless and odorless powder, which can be used in juices, cereals, cooked into breads, rolls or muffins, or taken with fruits or fruit juices, in order to help normalize the blood sugar after eating.

It must be pointed out that for the maximum improvement in the blood sugar to be realized, the glucomannan should be taken along with the meal which should include adequate quantities of fluid. The glucomannan only has its effect when properly hydrated by water.

The major impact of including glucomannan with meals is to reduce some of the symptoms of either elevated blood sugar or low blood sugar after meals; to sustain the release of glucose into the bloodstream and energy from the meal; to help improve blood fats by reducing cholesterol and triglyceride synthesis; and to encourage appetite suppression by increasing the volume of food in the stomach. The major difficulty with the use of glucomannan will be to insure its acceptance and palatability. The therapeutic dose generally used is between two to three teaspoons per meal. Some people find this difficult to tolerate, if the glucomannan is not properly combined with palatable foods.

Again, it should be recognized that glucomannan is an accessory food substance and not an essential nutrient. It is used for the therapeutic needs in people who have blood fat problems, are looking for appetite suppression or are trying to normalize blood sugar, and it falls nicely into the family of the accessory nutrients.

SUMMARY

The four accessory food factors we have discussed are representative of the explosion of information that is occurring in this branch of therapeutic nutrition. As more and more principles from various foods are concentrated and shown to have clinical response in certain individuals with needs determined by their own individual biochemistry, this field of therapeutic nutrition will grow ever more important.

All in all, these accessory food factors frame a class of substances that may prove vital for certain individuals in making the most of their health and wellness and serving as a useful adjunct to an improved diet. The thrust of the research indicates clearly that what is optimal nutrition for one may not be for another and that essential nutrients may be different from individual to individual, based upon the needs of each one. Octacosanol, carnitine, taurine and glucomannan are four representative examples of these substances which may prove some degree of "essentiality" for optimal health in a specific individual. This field of therapeutic nutrition will continue to explode with major health improvement resulting from this research.

REFERENCES

1. Spiller, G.A. 1982. Nutritional Pharmacology volume 4, in *Current Topics in Nutrition and Disease*. New York: Alan Liss, Inc.

2. Bessman, S.P. 1979. *Nutrition Reviews* 37, 209-211.

3. Spiller, G.A. 1980. *American Journal of Clinical Nutrition* 33, 1716-1719.

4. Smiley, W.A. 1951. Variations on a bicycle ergometer test with altitude, training, and a dietary supplement. M.S. thesis. University of Illinois.

5. White, C.H. 1951. The effect of physical training and a dietary supplement on the six Schneider index tests. M.S. thesis. University of Illinois.

6. Ershoff, B.A., and Levin, E. 1955. *Federation Proceedings* 14, 431-437.

7. Dukelow, W.R. 1963. *Acta Endocrinologica* pp. 5-15.

8. Alfin-Slater, R.B. 1960. *Federation Proceedings* 19, 18-22.

9. Deuel, H.J. 1951. In *The Lipids*. New York: Wiley-Interscience p. 361; also see reference 1, pp. 31-72.

10. Cureton, T.K. 1958. *Med. Sportiva* 12, 259-263.

11. Farrell, P.R. 1965. Effects of octacosanol on conception and oxygen uptake in the white rat. M.S. thesis. Kansas State University.

12. Bicknell, F. 1940. *Lancet,* pp. 10-11.

13. Stone, S. 1941. *Journal of American Medical Association* 18, 310-312.

14. Bremer, J. 1977. *Trends in Biochemical Sciences* 2, 207-209.

15. McGarry, J.D. and Foster, D.W. 1975. *Proceedings National Academy Sciences* 72, 4385-4388.

16. Broquist, H.P. 1976. *Nutrition Reviews* 34, 289-293.

17. Cederblad, G. 1977. *Clinical Chem. Acta* 67, 207-212.

18. Borum, P.R. and Broquist, H.P. 1977. *Journal Nutrition* 107, 1209-1215.

19. Hulse, J.D., Ellis, S.R. and Henderson, L.M. 1978. *Journal of Biological Chemistry* 253, 1654-1659.

20. Borum, P. 1981. *Nutrition Reviews* 39, 385-390.

21. Engel, A.G. and Angelini, C. 1973. *Science* 179, 899-902.

22. Chapoy, P.R., Angelini, C. and Brown, W.J. 1980. *New England Journal of Medicine* 303, 1389-1394.

23. Maebashi, M; Sato, M.; Immura, A.; and Yoshinaga, K. 1978. *Lancet*, October 14.

24. Carroll, J.E.; Brooke, M.H.; Shumate, J.B.; and Janes, N.J. 1981. *American Journal of Clinical Nutrition* 34, 2693-2698.

25. Mitchell, M.E. 1978. *American Journal of Clinical Nutrition* 31, 645-659.

26. Hayes, K.C. and Sturman, J.A. 1981. *Annual Reviews of Nutrition* 1, 401-425.

27. Awapara, J. 1976. In *Taurine,* ed., R. Huxtable, A. Barbeau pp. 1-19.

28. Baskin, S.I. and Finney, C.M. 1979. *Sulfur-Amino Acids* 2, 1-18.

29. Grosso, D.S., Bressler, R. and Benson, B. 1978. *Life-Sciences* 22, 1789-1798.

30. McLardy, T. 1962. *Nature* 194, 300-302.

31. Gaull, G.E., Rassia, D.K. and Heinonen, K. 1977. *Journal Pediatrics* 90, 348-355.

32. Barbeau, A. and Butterworth, R.F. 1975. *Life Sciences* 17, 669-677.

33. Thurston, J.H., Hauhart, R.E. and Naccarato, E.F. 1981. *Science* 214, 1373-1374.

34. Feldman, J. 1980. *Obesity and Bariatric Medicine* 9, 12-16.

35. McCallum, A.B. and Divertz, C. 1942. *Canadian Chemical Process Industry* 26, 569-570.

36. Gruener, R. and Huxtable, R. 1975. *Journal of Neurological Sciences* 24, 351-360.

37. Harrell, R.F., Capp, R.H. and Davis, D.R. 1981. *Proceedings National*

Academy of Sciences 78, 574-578.

38. Orlando, L.S. 1980. *Osteopathic Medicine* pp. 37-39.

39. Leichter, S. 1979. *American Journal of Clinical Nutrition* 32:2104-2114.

40. Anderson, J.W. and Ward, K. 1979. *American Journal of Clinical Nutrition* 32:2312-2321.

41. Jenkins, D. and Taylor, R. 1979. *Lancet* pp. 924-926.

42. Goulder, T.J. 1979. *Lancet* p. 617.

43. Doi, K. and Matsuura, M. 1979. *Lancet* pp. 987-988.

KEATS GOOD HEALTH GUIDES

25 Titles in Print or Preparation. . .

$1.45 per copy
Editors: Richard A. Passwater, Ph.D. and
Earl Mindell, R.Ph., Ph.D.

- **Aloe Vera, Jojoba and Yucca** by John Heinerman
- **Ask Jeanne Rose**
- **Brewer's Yeast, Wheat Germ and Other High Power Foods** by Beatrice Trum Hunter
- **Choline, Lecithin, Inositol and Other "Accessory" Nutrients Vol. 1** by Jeffrey Bland, Ph.D.
- **EPA—Marine Lipids** by Richard A. Passwater, Ph.D.
- **Evening Primrose Oil** by Richard A. Passwater. Ph.D.
- **First Aid With Herbs** by John Heinerman
- **GTF Chromium** by Richard A. Passwater, Ph.D.
- **Herbs and Herbal Medicine** by William H. Lee, R.Ph., Ph.D.
- **Hypoglycemia** by Marilyn Light
- **Lysine, Tryptophan and Other Amino Acids** by Robert Garrison, Jr., R.Ph., M.A.
- **Nutrition and Exercise for the Over 50s** by Susan Smith Jones
- **Nutrition and Stress** by Harold Rosenburg, M.D.
- **A Nutritional Guide for the Problem Drinker** by Ruth Guenther, Ph.D.

- **A Nutritional Guide for Women's Problems** by Nikki Goldbeck
- **Nutritional Parenting** by Sara Sloan
- **Octacosanol, Carnitine and Other "Accessory" Nutrients Vol. 2** by Jeffrey Bland, Ph.D.
- **Spirulina** by Jack Joseph Challem
- **A Stress Test for Children** by Jerome Vogel, M.D.
- **Tofu, Tempeh, Miso and Other Soyfoods** by Richard Leviton
- **Vitamin B3 (Niacin)** by Abram Hoffer, M.D., Ph.D.
- **Vitamin C Updated** by Jack Joseph Challem
- **Vitamin E Updated** by Len Mervyn, Ph.D.
- **The Vitamin Robbers** by Earl Mindell, Ph.D., R.Ph.
- **Wheat, Millet and Other Grains** by Beatrice Trum Hunter